LIP ENHANCEMENT PROCEDURES FOR BEGINNERS

Comprehensive Guide To Safe And Effective Techniques, Injections, Fillers, And Recovery Tips For Optimal Results

DR SAWYER DIEGO

DISCLAMER

Nothing in this book should be interpreted as medical advice; it is meant exclusively for educational reasons. Regarding their specific health issues and treatment options, readers are urged to speak with licensed healthcare professionals. The publisher and author disclaim all liability for any errors or omissions in the material provided, as well as for any negative effects that may arise from using or abusing the information. Although every attempt has been taken to guarantee that the material in this book is correct as of the date of publishing, new research may have superseded some of the content because medical knowledge is always changing. It is recommended that readers confirm the most recent medical recommendations and guidelines. The reader of this book undertakes to release the author and publisher from any claims or liabilities resulting from the use of this information, and understands and accepts the inherent risks connected with healthcare decisions.

TABLE OF CONTENTS

ABOUT THE BOOK

With a thorough introduction, the book lays the groundwork by explaining the complex anatomy of the lips, giving an overview of various lip enhancement techniques, and highlighting the significant benefits these procedures can offer. Readers will also learn how to properly prepare for lip enhancement as well as the vital aftercare and recovery tips necessary to achieve optimal results. Lip Enhancement Procedures for Beginners is an indispensable resource for anyone interested in learning about and exploring the world of lip enhancement.

This comprehensive approach guarantees that readers are well-informed about their options and the potential outcomes. The book explores the growing popularity and trends in the field, helping readers understand the goals of lip enhancement and how to choose the right procedure for their individual needs. It delves into the history of lip enhancement, tracing its evolution and highlighting the different types of procedures available today.

Dermal fillers for lip enhancement is one of the book's main topics; it describes the different kinds of dermal fillers, how they function, and the step-by-step process that goes along with them. The book also goes into great detail about the advantages, risks, and side effects of using dermal fillers, giving readers a well-rounded understanding of this natural augmentation method. Finally, the book discusses fat transfer lip enhancement in detail, outlining the procedure's benefits, potential risks, and recovery time, giving readers a comprehensive understanding of this natural augmentation method.

To help readers make an informed decision, the book also explores non-invasive lip enhancement options such as lip plumping devices, topical enhancers, and laser treatments. For those seeking a more permanent solution, it provides insights into lip implants, including the types available, the procedure itself, benefits, risks, and long-term care requirements.

For lip enhancement to be successful, selecting a qualified practitioner is essential. The book offers advice on what qualifications to look for, what to ask during consultations, and how to evaluate a practitioner's experience and expertise. It also emphasizes the value of comparing before and after photos and comprehending the consultation process to help readers make the best decision possible.

While aftercare and recovery are equally important, the book provides detailed advice on immediate post-procedure care, managing swelling and bruising, activity restrictions, and recognizing when to seek medical attention. Long-term care tips are also included to maintain the results. For those considering lip enhancement procedures, preparation is covered in detail, including advice on what to expect on the day of the procedure, what to avoid, and necessary lifestyle adjustments.

To give readers a comprehensive resource, common concerns, and frequently asked questions are addressed, including managing pain and discomfort, comprehending the longevity of results, and striking a balance between a natural look and enhanced features. Allergic reactions, sensitivities, and cost considerations are also covered.

This comprehensive approach guarantees that readers have all the information they need to achieve and sustain their desired lip enhancement results. Lastly, the book discusses how to maintain and enhance the results of lip enhancement procedures. It highlights the significance of follow-up appointments, touch-up procedures, a good skincare and lip care routine, healthy lifestyle choices, and recognizing and addressing any complications that may arise.

CHAPTER ONE

LIP ENHANCEMENT PROCEDURES OVERVIEW

KNOWING THE ANATOMY OF THE LIPS

Understanding the anatomy is essential for any lip enhancement procedure, as it helps practitioners avoid complications and achieve natural-looking results. The lips are a complex and delicate part of the human body, consisting of multiple layers and structures that contribute to their function and appearance. The outermost layer is the skin, which is thinner on the lips than elsewhere on the face, making them more sensitive. Beneath the skin is a layer of connective tissue that houses blood vessels, which give the lips their characteristic red color.

The lips are divided into two main sections: the upper lip and the lower lip. The upper lip has a characteristic curve called the Cupid's bow, which is often enhanced in cosmetic procedures. The lower lip is typically fuller and more prominent. The lips work in tandem with the surrounding muscles of the mouth to facilitate speaking, eating, and making facial expressions. Another important area that can be enhanced for a more defined appearance is the vermillion border.

A thorough understanding of these anatomical features is essential for performing lip enhancements safely and effectively, ensuring that the desired aesthetic results are achieved without compromising function. The inner structure of the lips includes the orbicularis oris muscle, which encircles the mouth and allows for movements such as puckering and smiling. The mucous membrane keeps the lips moist.

AN OVERVIEW OF TECHNIQUES FOR ENHANCING LIPS

There is a wide range of lip enhancement techniques that can be used to suit a variety of needs and preferences. One of the most common techniques is the use of injectable fillers, which are made of hyaluronic acid and give the lips volume and shape.

The procedure is minimally invasive and results can last for several months. The fillers can be precisely injected to achieve a desired look, whether it's a subtle enhancement or a more dramatic change.

Another popular procedure is lip implants, which offer a permanent solution for people who want volume that lasts. Made of soft, pliable materials like silicone, implants are inserted through small incisions at the corners of the mouth and require surgery but have a more durable result than fillers. Another surgical option is lip lifts, which involve removing a small amount of skin from just below the nose to elevate and reshape the upper lip.

Temporary improvements can be achieved with non-surgical methods like topical products and lip-plumping devices.

These methods are helpful for people who want a quick boost without committing to more invasive procedures. Each technique has pros and cons, so people need to speak with a qualified practitioner to figure out which is best for their unique goals and anatomy.

THE ADVANTAGES OF LIP AUGMENTATION PROCEDURES

The ability to create fuller, more youthful-looking lips is one of the main advantages of lip enhancement procedures. As we age, our lips naturally lose definition and volume, which makes them appear thinner. Enhancements can restore this lost volume, smooth out wrinkles around the mouth, and improve overall facial harmony.

Beyond the physical modifications, lip augmentations can greatly increase self-confidence. Many people experience self-consciousness regarding their lips, whether because of asymmetry, natural thinness, or age-related changes.

Improving the lips can make people feel more attractive and confident, which positively impacts their social interactions and self-esteem.

The changes in appearance can have a substantial impact on how people view themselves and are perceived by others.

Furthermore, the customized nature of lip enhancement procedures allows for individualized results. Surgeons can customize the treatments to match the patient's desired look, whether the patient is going for a more dramatic transformation or a subtle enhancement.

This flexibility guarantees that the results meet the patient's personal aesthetic goals, which gives the patient satisfaction and a sense of empowerment. Furthermore, the procedures are safer and more effective than ever thanks to advancements in techniques and materials.

GETTING READY FOR A LIP AUGMENTATION

A comprehensive consultation with a qualified practitioner is the first step towards ensuring the best possible outcome from a lip enhancement procedure.

The practitioner will evaluate the patient's lip anatomy, talk about the patient's aesthetic goals, and go over the various available enhancement options. They will also go over the patient's medical history and identify any potential risks or contraindications.

Practitioners may provide specific pre-procedure instructions, such as avoiding alcohol and smoking, which can affect healing and results. It is also advisable to avoid certain medications and supplements in the weeks leading up to the procedure, such as aspirin, ibuprofen, and vitamin E. Staying hydrated and maintaining good overall health can also help prepare the body for the procedure.

Wearing comfortable clothing and making arrangements for someone to drive them home, if necessary, can also help ensure a smooth experience. Having a clean face free of makeup and skincare products on the day of the procedure can help ensure a safer procedure and more satisfying results, setting the stage for a successful lip enhancement journey.

TIPS FOR RECOVERY AND AFTERCARE

Following lip enhancement surgery, some swelling, bruising, and tenderness are normal. Applying ice packs to the treated area can help reduce swelling and discomfort.

It's also important to avoid strenuous activities and excessive facial movements for the first few days to allow the lips to heal properly. Proper aftercare is essential to ensuring long-lasting results and minimizing complications.

Professionals may provide specific aftercare instructions, such as the use of any prescribed ointments or medications. Keeping the lips moisturized with a gentle, non-irritating balm can help in the healing process. Drinking plenty of water and staying hydrated will support overall recovery. Hot beverages, spicy foods, and alcohol are generally advised to avoid for at least 24 hours following the procedure, as these can exacerbate swelling and irritation.

Following up with the practitioner and letting them know about any concerns or unusual symptoms can help ensure that the results of a lip enhancement procedure are optimized and that the patient can confidently enjoy their enhanced appearance. Follow-up appointments are often scheduled to monitor the healing process and assess the results.

CHAPTER TWO
OVERVIEW OF LIP ENHANCEMENT

THE BACKGROUND OF LIP ENHANCEMENT

Lip enhancement procedures have a long history that dates back to ancient civilizations. Originally, lip enhancement was primarily used for cosmetic purposes; women in ancient Egypt would highlight their lips with natural dyes and henna. As time went on, techniques changed, and in the early 20th century, advances in medicine introduced surgical methods for lip augmentation. In the 1960s and 1970s, silicone injections were developed, but these were eventually abandoned due to complications.

Collagen injections gained popularity in the late 20th century as a safer and more effective way to increase lip volume. Hyaluronic acid fillers revolutionized the industry in the early 2000s with their natural results, minimal downtime, and safety profile. Regulatory bodies quickly approved these fillers, making them the preferred option for many people looking to enhance their lips.

The historical journey of lip enhancement highlights the importance of innovation and safety in cosmetic procedures.

Today, lip enhancement is a popular cosmetic procedure that people all over the world embrace. The evolution of techniques and materials over centuries reflects a continuous quest for safer, more natural-looking results.

TYPES OF PROCEDURES FOR LIP ENHANCEMENT

Several lip enhancement procedures can be chosen to suit a variety of needs and preferences. The most popular non-surgical option is the use of hyaluronic acid fillers, like Juvederm and Restylane, which are injected into the lips and provide temporary volume that can be adjusted to achieve desired results. The procedure is quick—it can be finished in as little as 30 minutes—and requires little recovery time.

In addition to hyaluronic acid fillers, lip grafting—a popular technique that involves harvesting fat from another part of the patient's body and injecting it into the lips—offers a more natural feel and longer-lasting results. Surgical options include lip implants, which involve permanently enhancing the lips with soft silicone implants; although this method offers long-term results, it requires a more involved procedure and recovery period.

By removing a small amount of skin from beneath the nose, lip lifts are a surgical option that changes the shape and position of the lips and gives a more youthful appearance by shortening the distance between the nose and the upper lip.

Since each of these procedures has advantages and disadvantages of its own, people need to speak with a qualified professional to find the procedure that best suits their needs.

TRENDS AND POPULARITY

Social media, celebrity culture, and advances in cosmetic technology have all contributed to the recent surge in the popularity of lip enhancement procedures. Open sharing of influencers' and celebrities' experiences and outcomes on platforms like Instagram and TikTok has helped normalize cosmetic enhancements and encouraged more people to research their options by lowering the stigma associated with them.

The current trend in lip enhancement is natural-looking enhancements that improve the volume and shape of the lips without looking too done.

The "Russian lip technique," which focuses on creating a defined cupid's bow and vertical lip height, is one technique that has gained popularity due to its aesthetically pleasing and natural results. Trends in lip enhancement often reflect broader beauty standards and cultural shifts.

Furthermore, there is a growing need for minimally invasive procedures that have short recovery times. Hyaluronic acid fillers are a popular choice because of their safety, reversibility, and customizable results. The trend toward customized cosmetic treatments guarantees that people can attain the look they want without sacrificing their natural appearance.

OBJECTIVES OF LIP ENHANCEMENT

The main objective of lip enhancement is to make the lips look better—fuller, more symmetrical, and more attractive. For many people, this means enhancing the overall attractiveness of the smile, making a more balanced facial profile, and adding volume to thin lips. Age-related changes, like lip thinning and the appearance of fine lines around the mouth, can also be addressed with lip enhancement.

Enhancing the lips can significantly improve self-esteem and body image, allowing people to feel more at ease and confident in their appearance. In addition, many people feel self-conscious about their lips because of their natural shape or changes over time.

Modern lip enhancement techniques are flexible enough to meet individual goals, so procedures can be customized to meet patient expectations and vision. Lip enhancement can also address specific aesthetic desires, such as defining the lip contours, creating a pronounced cupid's bow, or achieving a more youthful look.

SELECTING THE BEST PROCESS FOR YOU

Selecting the best lip enhancement procedure requires careful consideration of several factors, such as individual aesthetic goals, financial constraints, and the amount of downtime that the patient is willing to tolerate. It is important to understand the options that are available to you and choose the best course of action. A qualified cosmetic professional will examine the patient's lip anatomy, go over desired results, and make recommendations for appropriate procedures during the consultation.

Hyaluronic acid fillers are a great non-surgical option for people who want quick results with little downtime because they are flexible enough to allow for any necessary adjustments or reversals. If you're looking for something more permanent, lip implants or fat grafting might be suggested, but these require more involved procedures and longer recovery times.

The experience and expertise of the practitioner should also be taken into account. Selecting a competent and trustworthy expert can have a big impact on the procedure's safety and outcome. By doing their homework and talking with a qualified professional, people can make decisions that suit their needs and expectations and guarantee pleasing, natural-looking results.

CHAPTER THREE
DERMAL FILLERS TO BOOST LIPS
KINDS OF FILLERS IN THE SKIN

Dermal fillers come in a variety of forms, each intended to target different issues and facial regions. The most well-known type is hyaluronic acid (HA) fillers, which are renowned for their capacity to hydrate and add volume to the skin. Because of their reversibility and natural-looking results, HA fillers are frequently used for lip enhancement. Another popular type is calcium hydroxylapatite (CaHA) fillers, which offer a thicker, more substantial volume and are usually used for deeper lines and facial contouring. Polylactic acid (PLLA) fillers are also used to stimulate collagen production over time, providing longer-lasting results for facial volume loss.

Apart from these, there are also semi-permanent fillers called polymethyl methacrylate (PMMA) fillers, which are made up of small microspheres suspended in collagen gel; these are frequently used for deeper wrinkles and skin folds. Different types of dermal fillers have different properties, which makes them appropriate for different aesthetic goals. The area to be treated, the desired result, the patient's skin type, and overall health all play a role in the filler selection process.

Each filler type requires specific injection techniques, highlighting the importance of professional expertise in achieving optimal results. Being aware of the differences between these fillers helps beginners make informed decisions about their lip enhancement procedures. Speaking with a qualified practitioner is crucial to determining the most appropriate type of filler based on individual needs and expectations.

THE OPERATION OF DERMAL FILLERS

Dermal fillers plump up the skin by adding volume and fullness, which effectively reduces wrinkle appearance and enhances facial features. Hyaluronic acid fillers plump up the skin by attracting and holding onto water, which is a naturally occurring substance in the body that is safe and biocompatible to use in cosmetic procedures. Once injected, the filler becomes part of the skin, giving the skin a natural appearance and feel.

Polylactic acid fillers also stimulate collagen production, but they do so over a longer period, offering subtle, progressive results that improve with each treatment session. Calcium hydroxylapatite fillers, on the other hand, work differently by providing structural support and stimulating collagen production.

The microspheres in these fillers act as a scaffold, encouraging the body to produce collagen around them. This results in a gradual and natural enhancement that can last longer than HA fillers.

Understanding how each type of dermal filler works helps patients choose the right product for their specific needs, ensuring satisfactory and long-lasting results from their lip enhancement procedures.

Polymethyl methacrylate fillers are frequently used for more permanent correction of facial imperfections. These fillers provide immediate volume and stimulate collagen production, offering both short- and long-term benefits.

STEPS IN THE PROCEDURE

To minimize discomfort, the area surrounding the lips is cleaned and numbed with a topical anesthetic on the day of the procedure. Some fillers also contain lidocaine, a local anesthetic, which helps reduce pain during the injection process. The practitioner then marks the areas to be treated, ensuring precise and symmetrical results. The procedure for dermal fillers typically begins with a consultation where the practitioner assesses the patient's facial anatomy and discusses their aesthetic goals.

A tiny needle or cannula is used to carefully inject the filler into the desired areas; the technique varies based on the type of filler and the desired result. For lip enhancement, the filler is typically injected inside the lips to add volume and along the lip border to define the shape. The filler may be gently massaged into the targeted areas to ensure even distribution and to help shape the filler.

Follow-up appointments may be scheduled to assess results and make necessary adjustments. After injections, patients are usually able to resume normal activities with minimal downtime; swelling and bruising are common but usually go away within a few days. The practitioner provides aftercare instructions, which usually include avoiding strenuous activities, excessive sun exposure, and certain medications that can increase the risk of bruising.

ADVANTAGES OF INJECTABLE FILLERS

Dermal fillers are a popular option for lip augmentation because they provide several advantages over surgery. Firstly, patients can observe the results of the treatment immediately following the procedure, with lips appearing fuller and more defined. This immediate gratification is especially appealing to those who want to improve their appearance in a timely and efficient manner.

Dermal filler treatments also have the advantage of having minimal recovery time; unlike surgery, patients can resume their daily activities almost immediately after receiving a filler treatment; additionally, because the procedure is non-invasive, there are fewer risks and complications, making it a safer option for many people; and finally, most filler treatments have temporary effects that last between six months and two years, allowing for future adjustments and changes as needed.

Overall, dermal fillers provide a versatile, effective, and relatively low-risk solution for enhancing the lips and achieving a more youthful, balanced appearance. Practitioners can also customize the approach to lip enhancement with dermal fillers, ensuring natural-looking results. The ability to gradually build and adjust the volume over multiple sessions allows for greater precision and satisfaction.

HAZARDS AND ADVERSE REACTIONS

Although dermal fillers are considered safe in most cases, there are some risks and side effects that patients should be aware of. Bruising, swelling, and redness at the injection sites are common side effects that usually go away in a few days. Some patients may also experience tenderness or discomfort, which can be treated with cold compresses and over-the-counter pain relievers.

It is crucial to adhere to aftercare instructions to minimize these effects and guarantee appropriate healing.

More serious but uncommon side effects include vascular occlusion, allergic reactions, and infections. An allergic reaction can be itchy, rash, or swollen and necessitates immediate medical attention. An infection can result from improper sterilization of the injection site, causing redness, pain, and pus formation. Vascular occlusion is the result of the filler accidentally getting injected into a blood vessel, which can cause tissue damage and possibly result in skin necrosis or blindness.

A successful outcome can be ensured by adhering to all pre- and post-procedure guidelines, keeping open communication with the practitioner, and minimizing the risk of asymmetry or lumps forming under the skin. These issues can often be corrected with additional treatments or, in the case of hyaluronic acid fillers, with an enzyme called hyaluronidase that dissolves the filler.

CHAPTER FOUR

LIP ENHANCEMENT WITH FAT TRANSFER

FAT TRANSFER: WHAT IS IT?

In the context of lip enhancement, fat is typically harvested from areas like the abdomen, thighs, or buttocks, where there is an ample supply. This harvested fat is then purified and meticulously injected into the lips to create a fuller, more defined appearance. This method is preferred for its natural results, as the body's fat cells are used, reducing the risk of allergic reactions or rejection. Fat transfer, also known as fat grafting or lipofilling, is a cosmetic procedure that involves removing fat from one area of the body and injecting it into another area to enhance volume and shape.

Because the transferred fat integrates with the existing tissues, the results tend to be long-lasting, although some resorption of the fat may occur over time.

The main objective of fat transfer lip enhancement is to achieve a subtle, natural look that complements the individual's facial features. The procedure can be tailored to meet the specific desires of the patient, whether they seek a slight enhancement or a more dramatic change.

In addition to improving lips, fat transfer has the added benefit of contouring the donor site, which makes it a desirable procedure for people who want to improve their overall body shape. This technique is adaptable and can be used not only for lips but also for other areas that need volume restoration, like the hands, buttocks, and cheeks.

STEPS IN THE PROCEDURE

A consultation is required before beginning the fat transfer lip enhancement procedure, during which the surgeon evaluates the patient's suitability and discusses their desired aesthetic outcome. After a plan has been established, liposuction is used to harvest fat from the designated donor area; local anesthetic or sedation is applied to ensure patient comfort; the fat is carefully extracted using a small cannula by the surgeon, who then processes it to remove any impurities, leaving behind pure fat cells ready for injection.

Next, the surgeon carefully shapes the lips by strategically injecting the purified fat into various layers of the lip tissue with a fine needle, ensuring even distribution and results that look natural. This step requires a high level of precision and expertise to avoid overfilling and to achieve the desired symmetry and shape. The amount of fat injected is gradually built up.

Patients can usually see an immediate improvement in the fullness and shape of their lips, though some swelling and bruising are expected in the first few days after the procedure. After the injections, the treated areas are gently massaged to ensure the fat is distributed evenly. Depending on the extent of the enhancement, the procedure typically takes one to two hours. Detailed aftercare instructions are provided to ensure optimal healing and results.

BENEFITS OF TRANSFERRING FAT

Fat transfer is a safer alternative to synthetic fillers because it uses the patient's fat, which reduces the risk of allergic reactions or rejection. It also usually results in smoother, more natural-looking results that blend in seamlessly with the patient's existing lip tissue.

Finally, the longevity of fat transfer is a significant benefit because, although some of the transferred fat may be reabsorbed by the body, the remaining fat cells usually establish a permanent presence, providing long-lasting results.

Fat transfer has two advantages: it can improve body proportions and overall aesthetics by contouring the donor site during liposuction. It also provides a comprehensive solution for those who want to enhance their lips and address areas of excess fat.

The use of natural fat also removes concerns about foreign substances in the body, which can be especially appealing to those who are looking for a more holistic approach to cosmetic enhancement.

The ability to gradually build up the lips over multiple sessions, if necessary, also allows for incremental adjustments and fine-tuning of the results. Moreover, fat transfer enables greater customization in lip enhancement. Surgeons can precisely control the amount and placement of fat to achieve the desired volume and shape. This level of control enables a tailored approach, accommodating the unique needs and preferences of each patient.

DANGERS AND THINGS TO THINK ABOUT

Fat transfer for lip enhancement has many benefits, but there are risks involved as well. For example, the transferred fat may absorb unevenly, resulting in lumps or asymmetry that may require additional procedures to correct. Moreover, because part of the injected fat will be reabsorbed by the body, the initial results may fade over time and require touch-up procedures to maintain the desired look.

As with any surgical procedure, there is a risk of bleeding and infection as well. To reduce these risks, patients should adhere to all pre-and post-operative care instructions.

Bruising and swelling are common side effects, but they usually go away in a few weeks. Fat embolism, a serious health risk that arises when fat enters the bloodstream and blocks blood vessels, can also occur in rare cases.

Those who smoke or have certain medical conditions may not be the best candidates for fat transfer because their bodies' ability to heal is impaired. A comprehensive consultation with a qualified surgeon is necessary to assess suitability and go over potential risks and benefits. Being aware of these factors enables patients to make well-informed decisions and realistic expectations for the procedure's outcome.

HEALING AND OUTCOMES

Following fat transfer lip enhancement, recovery usually entails a few days of rest. Bruising, swelling, and tenderness can occur in both the donor and recipient sites; these symptoms can be managed with cold compresses and prescribed medications; avoid strenuous activities and keep the head elevated to reduce swelling; most patients are back to normal activities in a week or so; however, full recovery may take several weeks as the swelling goes down and the final results become apparent.

While the initial results of the procedure are immediately apparent, the ultimate result may not manifest for several months.

This is because a portion of the transferred fat will be reabsorbed by the body naturally, and the remaining fat cells require time to integrate with the surrounding tissue. To ensure optimal results, follow-up consultations with the surgeon are necessary to monitor the healing process and address any concerns. In certain instances, extra fat transfer sessions may be suggested.

One of the main advantages of fat transfer is the longevity of the results. Although some resorption of the fat is anticipated, the remaining fat cells that survive the transfer process usually provide a lasting enhancement. Patients can experience fuller, more defined lips for many years with appropriate care. Retaining a healthy weight and lifestyle can also help the results last longer. Frequent follow-ups with the surgeon guarantee continued satisfaction and enable any touch-ups that may be required to maintain the desired appearance.

CHAPTER FIVE

LIP IMPLANTS

LIP IMPLANT TYPES

There are several types of lip implants, each with varying degrees of enhancement and feel. The two most common types are silicone implants and expanded polytetrafluoroethylene (ePTFE) implants. Patients who want a subtle enhancement often choose silicone implants because they are soft, flexible, and have a natural feel. Patients who want a more pronounced and permanent augmentation may choose ePTFE implants because they are more rigid. Finally, some patients may choose to have fat grafting, which involves injecting fat from another area of the body into the lips. This procedure can provide a natural appearance but may need several sessions to get the desired result.

It is important to understand the differences between these implants, including their feel, longevity, and potential for complications, to make an informed decision. Choosing the right type of lip implant depends on the individual's goals, the desired level of fullness, and the advice of a qualified cosmetic surgeon. During a consultation, the surgeon will assess the patient's facial structure, skin type, and personal preferences to recommend the most suitable implant type.

Patients can choose the best approach for their desired lip enhancement by being aware of the pros and cons of each type of implant, which includes the ability to remove silicone implants if necessary, the deeper integration of ePTFE implants into the tissue, the possibility of uneven results from fat grafting, which is less invasive but may require touch-ups over time.

OVERVIEW OF THE PROCEDURE

First, the surgeon makes small incisions at the corners of the mouth to gain access to the lips where the implants will be placed. For silicone or ePTFE implants, the surgeon creates a tunnel within the lip tissue to accommodate the implant. This precise placement is crucial for achieving a natural look and feel. The procedure for lip implants is usually performed under local anesthesia with or without sedation, depending on the patient's comfort level.

The procedure usually takes 30 minutes to an hour, and patients can usually return home the same day. After the implants are positioned, the surgeon checks to make sure they are symmetrical and properly aligned. This may involve slightly adjusting the implant's position to achieve the desired fullness and shape. After confirming the placement, the incisions are closed with sutures that will be removed or dissolved within a few days.

Following post-operative care instructions is essential for optimal healing and results. Recovery involves some swelling and bruising, which can be managed with ice packs and prescribed pain medication. Most patients can return to normal activities within a week, although it's important to avoid strenuous activities and excessive lip movement during the initial healing period. The final results become more apparent as the swelling subsides, usually within a few weeks.

THE ADVANTAGES OF LIP IMPLANTS

One of the main advantages of lip implants—which are a popular choice for people who wish to have fuller lips—is their permanent enhancement. Unlike temporary fillers, which require ongoing care, lip implants provide a long-lasting solution for thin or uneven lips. This permanence allows patients to enjoy their improved appearance without having to undergo repeated treatments.

Modern lip implants also have the advantage of having a natural appearance and feel. Thanks to advancements in implant materials and techniques, patients can now achieve results that look and feel natural. Whether they choose silicone or ePTFE implants, patients can anticipate soft, flexible lips that allow for natural expressions and movement. This seamless integration boosts self-esteem and makes patients feel better about their appearance.

The precise and customizable enhancement that lip implants offer is another advantage. Surgeons can customize the size and shape of the implants to match the patient's facial features and preferences, guaranteeing that every patient receives the most harmonious and flattering results possible. Additionally, because the procedure is minimally invasive and relatively quick, patients can experience significant improvements with little downtime and recovery.

HAZARDS AND DIFFICULTIES

Like any surgical procedure, lip implants carry some risks and complications. The most frequent one is infection, which can happen if the incisions are not properly cleaned after the procedure; patients are typically prescribed antibiotics to prevent this, and proper hygiene is important during the healing process. Another risk is implant rejection, which is a condition in which the body rejects the implant because it feels like a foreign object and tries to remove it, which can cause discomfort and possibly require the removal of the implant.

Patients may also experience changes in sensation, such as numbness or increased sensitivity, though these are often transient and resolve as the lips heal. Other complications can include asymmetry, where the implants do not align perfectly, resulting in uneven lips. This can sometimes be corrected with a minor adjustment procedure. Scar tissue formation around the implant is another possible issue, which can lead to firmness or unnatural texture in the lips.

Selecting a knowledgeable and experienced cosmetic surgeon is critical to minimizing these risks. Carefully following all pre-and post-operative instructions can also help reduce the likelihood of complications. Regular follow-up appointments are essential to monitor healing and address any issues promptly. Preoperative consultations should include a thorough discussion of the patient's medical history, expectations, and any potential concerns.

Monitoring the condition of the implants and the surrounding tissue is crucial to maintaining optimal results. Although lip implants are intended to be a permanent solution, they may occasionally need to be adjusted or replaced over time, especially if complications arise or the patient's aesthetic preferences change.

Long-term care for lip implants involves routine check-ups with the cosmetic surgeon to ensure the implants remain in good condition and the lips retain their desired appearance.

Sustaining good overall lip health also means shielding the lips from too much sun exposure, which can degrade the elasticity and appearance of the skin; using SPF lip balms and keeping the lips moisturized can help maintain the lips' appearance and feel; patients should also be aware of any changes in appearance or sensation and notify their surgeon right away to address any potential problems early.

Patients can prolong the life of their lip implants by adhering to these guidelines and keeping in regular contact with their healthcare provider. Patients should also refrain from engaging in any activities that could cause trauma to the lips, such as harsh handling or excessive pressure. Finally, maintaining a healthy lifestyle, which includes eating a balanced diet and quitting smoking, can also support the longevity of the implants.

CHAPTER SIX

NON-INVASIVE TECHNIQUES FOR LIP ENHANCEMENT

DEVICES FOR LIP PLUMPING

Using a lip-plumping device is simple and effective compared to invasive procedures. It works by temporarily increasing blood flow to the lips, making them look plumper. First, apply a hydrating balm to your lips.

Then, place the device over your lips and gently press it against your mouth to create a seal. Next, activate the suction mechanism by squeezing or pumping, and hold it there for a few seconds to a minute, depending on the device's instructions. Finally, repeat these steps a few times, being careful not to exert too much pressure to prevent discomfort or bruises.

Lip plumping devices are a popular choice for quick and temporary lip enhancement; however, regular use can produce more noticeable results over time.

It's important to follow the manufacturer's guidelines and not exceed the recommended usage to prevent damage to the delicate skin on your lips. After using the device, apply a nourishing lip balm or gloss to maintain the plumped look and keep your lips hydrated. These devices are portable and convenient.

Overall, lip-plumping devices are a non-invasive and cost-effective way to achieve fuller lips; however, some users may experience mild discomfort or temporary bruising. It's important to use the device correctly and avoid overuse. If you have sensitive skin or any pre-existing conditions, consult a healthcare professional before using a lip-plumping device.

TOPICAL LIP ENHANCERS

Apply topical lip enhancer directly to clean, dry lips; you may feel tingling as the product starts to work. Your lips will look fuller and more voluminous in a few minutes. Topical lip enhancers, like lip plumping glosses and balms, are popular non-invasive options for enhancing lip volume.

These products contain ingredients like hyaluronic acid, peppermint oil, or cinnamon, which stimulate blood flow and cause a temporary swelling effect.

Topical lip enhancers are great for special occasions or when you want a quick boost to your lips' appearance.

They usually have temporary effects that last a few hours, and reapplication throughout the day can help maintain the plumped look. Many of these products also contain moisturizing ingredients that help keep your lips hydrated and smooth, which improves the appearance of your lips overall.

Topical lip enhancers are a widely accessible and affordable option for people who want to improve their lips without committing to more permanent procedures. However, before using any product on your lips, it's important to test it on a patch as some people may be allergic to certain ingredients or experience sensitivity to them.

LASER PROCEDURES

A laser is directed at the lips, penetrating the skin's surface without causing damage, and the procedure is quick—often finished in 30 minutes—with little discomfort or downtime. Laser treatments for lip enhancement are a non-invasive method that uses focused light energy to stimulate collagen production in the lips. This process helps to plump the lips naturally and improve their texture and volume over time.

Reduced fine lines and enhanced lip color are just two of the advantages of laser treatments. The gradual and natural-looking enhancement of the lips is another benefit.

Since the procedure stimulates collagen production, the results can last longer than topical enhancers or plumping devices. Usually, multiple sessions are needed to achieve the desired results, with effects becoming more noticeable over time.

To determine whether laser treatment is right for you, it's important to speak with a qualified professional who will evaluate your skin type and lip structure to design a personalized treatment plan. Although most laser treatments are safe, some people may experience temporary redness or swelling after the procedure. Proper aftercare, such as moisturizing and limiting sun exposure, is crucial to ensure optimal results and maintain lip health.

CONS AND BENEFITS OF NON-INVASIVE TECHNIQUES

Many people find non-invasive lip enhancement methods appealing because they don't involve needles or surgery, which lowers the possibility of complications and makes the procedure less scary for people who are afraid of invasive procedures. Non-invasive options, like topical enhancers, laser treatments, and lip-plumping devices, also usually involve little to no downtime, allowing patients to get back to their regular activities right away.

But, there are some disadvantages to take into account: the effects of non-invasive procedures are typically transient, necessitating continual upkeep to maintain the desired appearance; topical enhancers have short-term effects, and even laser treatments, while more permanent, may need repeated sessions and touch-ups; additionally, depending on the technique employed and the sensitivity of the patient's skin, some people may experience mild side effects like bruising or irritation.

Consulting with a professional can help you understand the potential outcomes and choose the non-invasive method that best suits your needs. Although non-invasive methods offer convenience and a lower risk profile, they may not provide the same level of enhancement as more permanent procedures, such as dermal fillers or surgical augmentation. It's important to weigh the pros and cons of each non-invasive option as well as your personal preferences and lifestyle.

DURATION AND EFFICACY

Lip plumping devices give instant results by increasing blood flow to the lips, making them appear fuller; however, these results are temporary, usually lasting a few hours. Regular use can help maintain a more consistent appearance, but the enhancement is not permanent. The effectiveness and duration of non-invasive lip enhancement methods vary depending on the technique used and individual factors.

Aside from being convenient for temporary enhancement—perfect for events or everyday use—topical lip enhancers also provide quick results, with the plumping effect appearing minutes after application.

The duration of the effect is typically a few hours, requiring reapplication to maintain the desired look. The overall effectiveness can vary depending on the formulation of the product and the skin type of the user.

Through the stimulation of collagen production, laser treatments provide a more gradual and long-lasting enhancement that can last for months. The effectiveness of laser treatments is often superior to other non-invasive methods, offering a more natural and sustained improvement in lip volume and appearance; however, achieving and maintaining the best results requires commitment to multiple treatments and proper aftercare.

CHAPTER SEVEN
SELECTING AN EXPERIENCED PROFESSIONAL
QUALIFICATIONS TO LOOK FOR

You should always make sure that a practitioner you choose for lip enhancement is qualified by looking for certifications from reputable medical boards or institutions. You should also look for practitioners who have received specialized training in lip enhancement techniques as this shows that they are dedicated to mastering the procedure and staying up to date with the latest advancements. Licensed medical professionals, such as dermatologists, plastic surgeons, or certified aestheticians with specialized training in cosmetic procedures, are the best candidates for this type of work.

Membership in professional organizations in dermatology or cosmetic surgery is another crucial credential. Membership in organizations such as the American Society for Dermatologic Surgery or the

American Board of Cosmetic Surgery shows that the practitioner maintains high standards of practice and continuous education. These memberships frequently require practitioners to meet strict requirements and stay up to date with industry developments, ensuring they maintain the skills necessary to perform procedures safely and effectively.

Finally, take into account the practitioner's hospital privileges, which enable them to conduct procedures in surgical centers or accredited hospitals. Hospital affiliations serve as a safety net, guaranteeing that practitioners have access to cutting-edge medical resources and support if complications arise during or after the procedure. Hospital affiliations are a strong indicator of a practitioner's competency and reliability, as hospitals conduct thorough evaluations before granting privileges.

WHAT TO ASK IN A CONSULTATION

Find out during your consultation how long the practitioner has been doing lip enhancement procedures, how many procedures they perform annually, and how experienced they are with the procedure; these questions will help you determine the practitioner's level of experience and familiarity with different techniques and potential complications. You should also find out about the products they use, such as the type of fillers, and why they use them; knowing the products and their benefits will help you make an informed decision.

It's also critical to talk about possible risks and complications. Get information from the practitioner about potential side effects and how they manage them. You can feel more confident in their ability to provide safe care if you know how they handle complications like infections or allergic reactions. You should also ask about how long the results will last and if any maintenance procedures are needed to maintain the desired appearance.

To ensure you are well-prepared for the procedure, ask about any pre-and post-procedure care instructions to maximize your results and minimize recovery time. Lastly, ask for a detailed explanation of the procedure, including the steps involved, the expected duration, and the recovery process. Communicating clearly and providing thorough explanations are signs of a practitioner who prioritizes patient education and satisfaction.

EVALUATING KNOWLEDGE AND EXPERIENCE

To ensure that lip enhancement procedures are successful, you must assess the experience and expertise of the practitioner. Look for practitioners who have performed a significant number of lip enhancement procedures; this can be found by looking at how many procedures they have completed and how long they have been in practice. Experience is often associated with a higher level of skill and a better understanding of the subtleties involved in achieving results that look natural.

Inquire about their specific training in lip enhancement procedures.

Advanced-trained practitioners or those who frequently attend workshops and conferences are more likely to be knowledgeable about the newest techniques and technologies. Their continued education shows that they are dedicated to giving their patients the best possible results. You should also find out if they have any specialties or techniques that they prefer using, as this can give you an idea of their areas of expertise and ability to customize procedures to meet the needs of each individual.

In the end, a combination of experience, specialized training, and positive patient feedback will help you choose a practitioner who can deliver excellent lip enhancement results. Take into consideration their reputation and patient reviews. Look for testimonials or before-and-after photos that showcase their work. Positive reviews and visual evidence of successful procedures can help build trust in their abilities. Furthermore, word-of-mouth recommendations from friends or family who have undergone similar treatments can be invaluable in identifying a skilled and reliable practitioner.

THE VALUE OF BEFORE AND AFTER IMAGES

A practitioner's skill and the possible results of a lip enhancement procedure can both be evaluated by looking at before and after photos, which give you a visual representation of the practitioner's work and allow you to see real examples of their results. Additionally, photos should show a variety of cases, which highlights the practitioner's ability to customize treatments to different patient preferences and facial structures. Natural-looking volume, symmetry, and proportion are examples of enhancements that you should look for in a practitioner.

Looking at before and after photos can help you evaluate the practitioner's aesthetic compatibility with your desired outcome as well as their ability to achieve the subtlety and precision you seek.

You can evaluate the smoothness of the lip contour, the even distribution of filler, and the overall harmony with the patient's facial features. Quality results should enhance the lips while maintaining a natural appearance, avoiding an overfilled or artificial look.

Bringing examples of what you like and dislike to discuss with the practitioner also helps to ensure that you and the practitioner are on the same page regarding your expectations. Seeing concrete proof of the practitioner's prior work gives you confidence in their ability to deliver the results you want and helps you make an informed decision about moving forward with the treatment.

COMPREHENDING THE CONSULTATION PROCEDURE

A key component of organizing your lip enhancement procedure is the consultation process. In this consultation, the physician will review your medical history, current health status, and history of cosmetic procedures to evaluate your suitability for lip enhancement. This thorough assessment helps identify potential risks and confirms that you are a good candidate for the procedure. You should be prepared to go over your expectations and goals in detail as this will help the physician create a customized treatment plan.

The practitioner will assess your unique features during the consultation to customize the treatment to your desired results, ensuring a harmonious and natural enhancement. They will also go over the various techniques and products that are available to you, assisting you in understanding your options and making an informed decision. The practitioner will examine your facial anatomy, including the shape and symmetry of your lips, to recommend the best approach for achieving your desired results. They may take measurements or use digital imaging to visualize potential outcomes.

CHAPTER EIGHT

GETTING READY FOR YOUR LIP SCULPTING PROCESS

PRE-PROCEDURE GUIDELINES

Following specific pre-procedure instructions is essential to ensuring the best outcome and minimizing complications from your lip enhancement procedure.

To start, you should wash your face completely the day before the procedure so that the treated area is free of contaminants that could cause infections. You should also drink plenty of water in the days before to keep your skin in the best possible condition.

Apart from that, stay away from any physically demanding activities that could enhance blood flow to your face, like intense workouts or sauna sessions. These activities can worsen swelling and bruises after the procedure. You should also abstain from alcohol and tobacco for at least 48 hours before the procedure, as these can hurt the healing process and the procedure's overall result.

To help your practitioner selects the safest products and techniques for your particular needs, be sure to discuss any allergies or past reactions to anesthetics or fillers with them. Carefully following these pre-procedure instructions will help ensure a more seamless procedure and more satisfying results.

AVOIDING SUPPLEMENTS AND MEDICATIONS

Before your lip enhancement procedure, avoid taking certain medications and supplements as they can thin your blood and increase the chance of excessive bleeding and bruising. Nonsteroidal anti-inflammatory drugs (NSAIDs) like aspirin, ibuprofen, and naproxen should be stopped at least one week before your procedure.

Avoid supplements that thin the blood, such as fish oil, vitamin E, and ginkgo biloba. Natural remedies, like garlic, ginger, and turmeric, can also thin the blood; limit their use in your diet before the procedure. Tell your practitioner about everything you take, including vitamins and supplements, so they can give you specific advice on what to stop taking.

Appropriate management of your medication and supplement intake will help ensure a more straightforward procedure with few complications. If you are taking prescription blood thinners or any other necessary medication, speak with your healthcare provider before making any changes. Your safety is the most important thing, so professional guidance is required when making any changes.

MODIFICATIONS TO LIFESTYLE

Before your lip enhancement procedure, there are a few lifestyle changes that can greatly affect the healing process and final results. First and foremost, make sure you are eating a vitamin- and mineral-rich, well-balanced diet that will support your body's natural healing processes; include lots of fruits, vegetables, and lean proteins in your meals, but stay away from processed foods and sugary drinks.

In addition, getting enough sleep is essential. In the weeks preceding your procedure, try to get 7 to 8 hours of good sleep every night. This will help you recover better by boosting your immune system and lowering stress. You can also lower your stress levels by practicing yoga, meditation, or deep breathing exercises. Stress can hinder your body's natural healing process.

Finally, it is strongly advised that smokers give up at least two weeks before and following their procedure. Smoking can obstruct blood flow and considerably slow down the healing process, which may result in complications.

WHAT TO ANTICIPATE ON THE PROCEDURE DAY

Your practitioner will start by going over the procedure one last time and answering any last questions or concerns you may have.

On the day of your lip enhancement procedure, it's important to arrive calm and prepared. Wear comfortable clothing and make sure you've eaten a light meal a few hours before your appointment to keep your blood sugar levels stable.

When you're ready, a topical anesthetic will be applied to your lips to reduce any discomfort. This usually takes 20 to 30 minutes to take effect. Then, the practitioner will carefully administer the filler to your lips, enhancing their shape and volume. Depending on the complexity and extent of the enhancement, the entire procedure may take 30 to 60 minutes.

It's normal to experience some swelling and bruising, which should subside within a few days. Your practitioner will give you post-procedure care instructions and may apply an ice pack to help reduce swelling after the injections are finished. You will be able to see the initial results immediately, with the outcome becoming more apparent as the swelling reduces.

PSYCHOLOGICAL READINESS

To ensure that your lip enhancement procedure goes well, psychological preparation is essential. Start by establishing reasonable expectations for the outcome; realize that although the procedure can dramatically improve your appearance, it is not a miracle cure for deeper problems with self-esteem or body image; and be transparent with your practitioner about your concerns and goals so that you both know exactly what you hope to achieve.

It's crucial to control any anxiety or nervousness you may have in the days before the procedure. Try mindfulness exercises, meditation, or even light physical activity to help de-stress. Speaking with friends or family members who have had comparable procedures done can also reassure you and give you insight into what to expect.

Finally, schedule a day or two off work if feasible, and stock your home with comfort supplies like soft foods, ice packs, and entertainment.

CHAPTER NINE
RECUPERATION AND AFTERCARE
QUICK POST-PROCEDURE TREATMENT

Immediately following a lip enhancement procedure, apply ice packs to the treated area for 10-15 minutes at a time. This helps reduce swelling and provides some relief from discomfort. Be careful not to apply too much pressure, and always place a clean cloth or protective barrier between the ice pack and your skin to prevent frostbite. Following lip enhancement procedures, these specific aftercare steps are critical to ensuring optimal healing and results.

To keep your lips moisturized during the initial healing phase, use a gentle, non-irritating lip balm (avoid products with harsh chemicals or fragrances). Avoid touching or massaging your lips as this can introduce bacteria and increase the risk of infection. Drink plenty of water and avoid alcohol as it can cause dehydration and exacerbate swelling.

Attending all follow-up appointments is crucial to ensuring proper healing and addressing any concerns or complications that may arise. In addition, it's important to follow any specific instructions provided by your healthcare provider. These may include taking prescribed medications, such as antibiotics or pain relievers, to manage discomfort and prevent infection.

HANDLING BRUISING AND SWELLING

Following lip enhancement procedures, swelling and bruising are common side effects. To manage swelling, use ice packs on and off for the first 24 to 48 hours. When sleeping, elevate your head by using extra pillows; this can help reduce swelling by encouraging fluid to drain away from the treated area.

Avoiding drugs and supplements that thin the blood and increase the risk of bruising, such as aspirin, ibuprofen, and vitamin E, can help reduce bruising.

Natural remedies like arnica cream, which is often prescribed by medical professionals, can also help reduce bruising; gently apply the cream to the bruised areas as directed.

For a minimum of 48 hours following the procedure, refrain from physically demanding activities, hot showers, saunas, and sun exposure as these may intensify blood flow to the treated area, aggravating swelling and bruises. Should you experience unusual symptoms or bruising that lasts longer than a week, get in touch with your healthcare provider for additional assessment.

LIMITATIONS ON ACTIVITIES

Certain physical activities, such as heavy lifting, intense workouts, and any activity that raises your heart rate significantly, should be avoided for at least 48 to 72 hours after lip enhancement surgery to promote healing and prevent complications. These activities can increase blood flow and swelling, which could potentially impact the healing process.

For a week or more, avoid doing anything that puts pressure on your lips directly, like kissing. You should also refrain from getting facial massages or other lip-related treatments, as well as hot beverage and straw use, which can put strain on the area that has been treated.

To lower the chance of infection, it's also a good idea to refrain from applying makeup to the lips for at least 24 hours. When you do decide to wear makeup again, make sure all of the products and applicators are clean to prevent bringing bacteria into the healing lips. Finally, pay attention to your healthcare provider's advice regarding when it's safe to return to your regular activities.

WHEN TO GET MEDICAL HELP

After a lip enhancement procedure, it's critical to closely monitor your healing and know when to seek medical attention. If you experience intense or worsening pain that does not go away with prescribed medication, get in touch with your healthcare provider right away as this could be a sign of an infection or other complication that needs to be treated right away.

Infection symptoms include fever, chills, and flu-like symptoms; you should also report any signs of infection to your provider, such as excessive redness, warmth, swelling, or pus. If your bruises and swelling don't go better after a reasonable amount of time, you should see a doctor to rule out any complications.

Additionally, always err on the side of caution and get in touch with your healthcare provider if you have any concerns about your recovery or if you experience any symptoms that seem out of the ordinary. If you notice any signs of an allergic reaction, such as breathing difficulties, hives, or swelling in areas other than your lips, seek emergency medical attention.

TIPS FOR LONG-TERM CARE

Maintaining the results of your lip enhancement procedure and maintaining the health of your lips requires proper long-term care. You should use a high-quality lip balm regularly to prevent dryness and keep your lips hydrated. You should choose products with SPF to protect your lips from sun damage, which can negatively impact the appearance and health of the area that has been treated.

Keep up a healthy lifestyle by drinking plenty of water and eating a well-balanced diet high in vitamins and minerals, both of which promote good skin. Refrain from smoking and drink in moderation since these can wreak havoc on your lips' state and hasten the aging process.

Make routine follow-up appointments with your healthcare provider to discuss any concerns and assess the condition of your lips. They can offer professional advice on how to maintain your results and recommend touch-up treatments if needed.

CHAPTER TEN
FREQUENTLY ASKED QUESTIONS
RESOLVING PAIN AND UNEASE

Discussing pain management options with your practitioner will ensure a comfortable experience. When considering lip enhancement procedures, it's important to understand how pain and discomfort are managed. Most procedures, like injections, involve the use of numbing agents to minimize pain. Topical anesthetics are commonly applied to the lips before the procedure, numbing the area and significantly reducing the sensation of pain. Some practitioners also use ice packs or vibrating devices to further distract from the discomfort.

Following the procedure, patients may have mild bruising, soreness, and swelling. These side effects are usually transient, lasting only a few days. You can minimize discomfort by taking over-the-counter pain relievers like ibuprofen, and you can apply ice packs to help reduce swelling.

It's important to follow your practitioner's aftercare instructions to ensure a smooth recovery process. Additionally, keeping the treated area clean and avoiding strenuous activities for the first 24 hours can help speed up recovery.

Selecting a highly skilled and experienced practitioner is beneficial for those who are worried about pain, as their knowledge can expedite and lessen the discomfort of the procedure. Being open and honest about your concerns and pain tolerance allows the practitioner to adjust their approach and employ the best pain management techniques. This cooperative approach makes sure that the experience is as stress-free and comfortable as possible.

DURATION OF OUTCOMES

Dermal fillers, the most popular method, typically last between six months to a year. The exact product used, the amount injected, and how quickly the body metabolizes the filler all play a role in determining the duration of the results.

For more lasting outcomes, semi-permanent or permanent options like fat transfer or lip implants are available, though these come with their own set of considerations. The longevity of lip enhancement results varies depending on the type of procedure and the individual's metabolism.

In addition to scheduling touch-up appointments to maintain the desired volume and shape of your lips, maintenance treatments can help prolong the life of lip enhancements. Lifestyle choices like avoiding excessive sun exposure, quitting smoking, and adhering to a healthy diet can also help prolong the results of your enhancements. Speaking with your practitioner about the best maintenance routine can help you achieve long-lasting satisfaction with your enhanced lips.

While some people may experience longer-lasting effects, others may require more frequent touch-ups. Discussing your goals and lifestyle with your practitioner will help determine the most suitable type of enhancement and maintenance plan, ensuring you achieve and maintain your desired look over time. Knowing the expected timeline for results is important for managing expectations.

ENHANCED LOOK VS. NATURAL LOOK

One common concern among those who are thinking about lip enhancements is finding the right balance between an enhanced appearance and a natural look. A natural look seeks to improve the volume and shape of the lips while keeping them in harmony with the facial features. This can be accomplished by using smaller amounts of filler and concentrating on enhancing the natural contours of the lips. The objective is to create an appearance that is more youthful and refreshed without being overtly enhanced.

The choice between a natural and an enhanced look largely depends on personal preferences and aesthetic goals. Speaking with a skilled practitioner who understands your vision is essential for achieving the desired outcome.

For those seeking a more noticeable enhancement, larger volumes of filler can be used to create fuller, more defined lips. This approach can result in a more dramatic change, making the lips a focal point of the face.

Successful lip enhancement requires tailoring the procedure to each person's unique facial structure and desired outcomes. Advanced techniques, such as enhancing the Cupid's bow or adding definition to the vermillion border, can achieve the desired balance between natural and enhanced without overdoing the lips. It is important to communicate your expectations and preferences to your practitioner to ensure that the treatment plan is tailored to your needs and goals.

SENSITIVITIES AND ALLERGIC REACTIONS

As hyaluronic acid is a naturally occurring substance in the body, dermal fillers are generally well-tolerated; however, allergic reactions can still occur, especially with fillers that contain additional ingredients or preservatives. A thorough medical history review and possibly a patch test can help identify potential allergic reactions before proceeding with the treatment. You must discuss any known allergies or sensitivities with your practitioner before undergoing a lip enhancement procedure.

To reduce the risk of complications during the procedure, practitioners take precautions such as using reputable, high-quality filler brands and making sure that sterile techniques are followed. If an allergic reaction does occur, symptoms may include redness, swelling, itching, or even more severe reactions. To effectively manage such reactions, prompt medical attention and appropriate treatment are required. It is important to know the signs of an allergic reaction and how to respond.

Aftercare instructions from the practitioner, such as avoiding certain skincare products or places that might cause an allergic reaction, can help prevent problems. It's also important to stay hydrated and avoid excessive sun exposure, as these can exacerbate sensitivities. To ensure a safe and comfortable procedure, it's crucial to have open and honest communication with your practitioner before, during, and after the procedure.

EXPENSE FACTORS

The cost of lip enhancement procedures varies greatly depending on several factors, such as the type of procedure, the experience level of the practitioner, and the clinic's location. Dermal fillers are usually priced per syringe, and the total cost can vary from a few hundred to several thousand dollars, depending on the amount of filler required to achieve the desired result. It is crucial to obtain a detailed quote and understand what is included in the price, such as follow-up appointments or additional treatments if necessary.

Lower-cost options may compromise the quality of the product used or the practitioner's expertise, potentially leading to unsatisfactory results or complications.

Investing in a qualified practitioner ensures a higher standard of care and better overall outcomes. Cost is an important consideration, but it shouldn't be the only one. Selecting a highly experienced and reputable practitioner can significantly impact the safety and quality of the results.

A smooth and stress-free experience can be ensured by being aware of all the cost-related factors and making appropriate plans. Many clinics offer payment plans or financing options to make the procedure more affordable. It's worth discussing these options with your chosen clinic to find a plan that fits your budget. Additionally, some clinics might offer discounts for multiple treatments or referrals, making it easier to maintain the desired look without straining finances.

CHAPTER ELEVEN

SUSTAINING AND IMPROVING OUTCOMES

RESCHEDULED APPOINTMENTS

Following lip enhancement procedures, it's important to schedule follow-up appointments to monitor your progress and ensure optimal results. These appointments are usually scheduled a few weeks after the initial treatment and give your practitioner a chance to see how well your lips have responded to the enhancement and address any concerns you may have. Your practitioner will examine the symmetry, shape, and volume of your lips to see if any adjustments or touch-ups are needed, as well as to hear about your satisfaction with the results and offer advice on how to maintain your lip health.

Maintaining consistent follow-up visits ensures that your lip enhancement continues to meet your aesthetic goals and remains safe and effective over time.

Regular follow-up appointments also help to track the longevity of your lip enhancement. Your practitioner will advise you on when to consider future treatments based on how your body metabolizes the filler or if you opt for a semi-permanent procedure like fat transfer. You can ask questions about any changes you may notice in your lips and receive personalized advice on lip care during these appointments.

Attending follow-up appointments as advised shows your commitment to the procedure and your overall satisfaction with the improvements made to your lips. Good communication with your practitioner during these sessions is essential to achieving and maintaining satisfactory results from lip enhancement procedures.

TOUCH-UP TECHNIQUES

Touch-ups are usually scheduled during follow-up appointments based on your practitioner's assessment or at your request if you feel additional enhancement is necessary.

The goal of touch-up procedures is to ensure that your lips look natural and harmonious with your facial features, addressing any areas that may require further enhancement. Touch-ups are occasionally necessary to refine the results of your initial lip enhancement treatment. These procedures involve making minor adjustments to achieve the desired symmetry, volume, or shape of your lips.

Touch-up procedures are usually quick and involve minimal discomfort, similar to the initial treatment session. Your practitioner will use the same techniques as the initial treatment, whether it involves injecting additional filler or adjusting the existing filler for optimal results. They will discuss your expectations and desired outcomes beforehand to tailor the touch-up to your preferences.

Maintaining the longevity and appearance of your lip enhancements requires adhering to your practitioner's recommendations for touch-up procedures. You can achieve a balanced and natural-looking result that improves your overall facial aesthetics by addressing minor imperfections or asymmetries through touch-ups. Regular communication with your practitioner guarantees that touch-up procedures are performed safely and effectively, which adds to your satisfaction with the enhancement process.

ROUTINE FOR SKINCARE AND LIP CARE

A gentle skincare routine that includes moisturizing and shielding your lips from the sun can help preserve the volume and texture of your enhanced lips. Using products with hydrating ingredients like hyaluronic acid or shea butter can also help keep your lips smooth and supple. Creating a skincare and lip care routine is essential for maintaining the health and appearance of enhanced lips. After undergoing lip enhancement procedures, your lips may require specific care to ensure longevity and optimal results.

Applying lip balms or treatments that moisturize and shield your lips is the first step in incorporating a lip care routine into your daily routine.

Look for products that are designed to hydrate and condition, rather than harsh ingredients that could irritate your lips' delicate skin. Regular exfoliation can help remove dead skin cells and encourage circulation, which will improve the appearance of your lips after treatment.

Finally, wearing sunscreen on your lips when exposed to UV rays can help prevent premature aging and preserve the results of your enhancement.

Incorporating these practices into your daily routine will help you achieve and maintain beautiful, healthy lips that enhance your natural beauty. Speak with your practitioner or skincare specialist for personalized recommendations on products and techniques that best suit your skin type and lip enhancement goals. A healthy skincare and lip care routine also promotes overall lip health and prolongs the benefits of treatment.

CHOOSING A HEALTHIER LIFESTYLE

Supporting the outcomes of lip enhancement procedures and promoting overall well-being requires making healthy lifestyle choices. Lifestyle choices like eating a balanced diet, drinking plenty of water, and quitting smoking can have a big impact on how long your enhanced lips last and look.

A diet high in vitamins and antioxidants supports skin health, which includes the delicate skin on your lips, and drinking enough water keeps your lips volumized and texture intact.

Frequent exercise supports the long-term benefits of lip enhancement treatments by promoting circulation and enhancing the overall vitality of the skin, including the lips. Preserving the results of your enhancement over time can be achieved by avoiding excessive sun exposure and wearing sunscreen on your lips to prevent premature aging and protect against UV damage.

Stress can contribute to facial tension and affect the appearance of skin, including the lips. Managing your stress levels with mindfulness exercises or relaxation techniques can also improve the results of your lip enhancement procedure. You can support the appearance and general health of your lips after treatment by adopting healthy coping mechanisms and making self-care a priority. These lifestyle choices also extend the longevity of your lip enhancements and encourage a balanced, natural aesthetic that accentuates your facial features.

IDENTIFYING AND DEALING WITH ISSUES

Even though lip enhancement procedures are generally safe when carried out by a qualified practitioner, it's important to be aware of potential complications that could occur. Early signs of complications, like excessive swelling, persistent pain, or unusual changes in lip appearance, are important to recognize to ensure appropriate treatment and prevent further complications.

If you experience any concerning symptoms, get in touch with your practitioner right away.

Following post-procedure care instructions and attending follow-up appointments are essential for monitoring your recovery and addressing any complications as soon as they arise.

Common complications from lip enhancement procedures include allergic reactions to filler ingredients, infection at the injection site, or uneven distribution of filler causing asymmetry. Your practitioner can assess the severity of any complications and recommend appropriate measures, such as medications or corrective procedures, to address them effectively.

You may reduce risks and achieve safe, satisfactory results from lip enhancement procedures by educating yourself about potential risks and complications related to these procedures. Being watchful in identifying and resolving complications guarantees that your lip enhancement experience stays positive and effectively enhances your natural beauty. You can also reduce risks and take proactive steps in your care by keeping lines of communication open with your practitioner and promptly seeking medical attention for any concerns.